THE USER GUIDE TO
BREAST HEALTH

A COMPREHENSIVE GUIDE TO
BREAST HEALTH AND CANCER
AWARENESS

JULIANNA PARRA

Table of Contents

CHAPTER ONE

INTRODUCTION

Understanding Breast Anatomy

Understanding breast anatomy is fundamental to promoting breast health and raising awareness about breast cancer. The human breast is a complex organ consisting primarily of glandular tissue, ducts, adipose tissue (fat), and connective tissue. While often associated solely with lactation and nurturing offspring, the breast serves multifaceted roles in the body, including hormonal regulation and immune defense.

At its core, breast health encompasses the maintenance of optimal physiological function and the prevention, early detection, and treatment of breast-related diseases, with breast cancer being the most prevalent concern. Breast cancer is a heterogeneous disease characterized by the uncontrolled growth of abnormal cells in breast tissue. It can manifest in various forms, including invasive ductal carcinoma, invasive lobular carcinoma, and less common subtypes.

Understanding breast anatomy provides a foundation for comprehending the intricacies of breast cancer development and detection. The breast consists of fifteen to twenty lobes, each containing smaller lobules that produce milk during lactation. These lobules are interconnected by ducts, which transport milk to the nipple. Adipose tissue surrounds the lobules and ducts, providing support and cushioning. Additionally, an extensive network of blood vessels and lymphatic vessels traverses the breast, facilitating nutrient delivery and waste removal.

The significance of breast anatomy extends beyond its physiological structure to encompass the mechanisms underlying breast cancer initiation and progression. Breast cancer often originates in the epithelial cells lining the ducts or lobules, where genetic mutations can disrupt normal cellular processes, leading to unchecked proliferation. As the disease advances, cancerous cells may invade surrounding tissue and metastasize to distant organs, posing significant health risks.

Moreover, understanding breast anatomy is crucial for interpreting breast imaging modalities utilized in cancer screening and diagnosis. Techniques such as mammography, magnetic resonance imaging (MRI), and ultrasound rely on knowledge of breast composition and architecture to identify abnormalities indicative of malignancy. By recognizing the spatial relationships between different breast components, healthcare professionals can discern subtle changes suggestive of early-stage cancer.

Beyond pathology, understanding breast anatomy fosters appreciation for the diversity of breast shapes, sizes, and variations among individuals. Such awareness promotes inclusivity and sensitivity in discussions surrounding breast health, recognizing that norms and perceptions may differ across cultures and communities.

CHAPTER TWO

THE IMPORTANCE OF BREAST HEALTH

Breast health is a critical aspect of overall well-being, encompassing physical, emotional, and social dimensions. From nurturing infants through lactation to serving as symbols of femininity and self-identity, breasts play multifaceted roles in the lives of individuals. However, beyond their cultural and aesthetic significance, prioritizing breast health is paramount for early detection and prevention of breast cancer, a disease that affects millions worldwide each year.

Breast cancer is the most common cancer among women globally, with incidence rates varying across populations and regions. Despite advancements in screening and treatment, it remains a significant public health challenge, underscoring the importance of proactive measures to promote breast health. By cultivating awareness, fostering early detection, and advocating for comprehensive care, individuals can reduce their risk of developing breast cancer and improve treatment outcomes.

One of the primary reasons for emphasizing breast health is the potential to detect breast cancer in its early stages when treatment is most effective. Regular breast self-exams, clinical breast exams, and screening mammograms enable the identification of abnormalities such as lumps, changes in breast size or shape, or skin dimpling. Early detection facilitates prompt intervention, including diagnostic testing and treatment initiation, thereby increasing the likelihood of successful outcomes and reducing mortality rates.

Moreover, prioritizing breast health empowers individuals to adopt proactive lifestyle choices that may lower their risk of developing breast cancer. Factors such as maintaining a healthy weight, engaging in regular physical activity, limiting alcohol consumption, and avoiding tobacco use have been linked to reduced breast cancer risk. Additionally, breastfeeding and hormone replacement therapy decisions can influence breast health outcomes, highlighting the importance of informed decision-making and preventive measures.

Beyond physical health, breast health encompasses emotional and psychosocial well-being, acknowledging the impact of breast cancer diagnosis and treatment on individuals and their families. Fear, anxiety, and uncertainty are common emotional responses to a breast cancer diagnosis, underscoring the need for comprehensive support services and survivorship care. By addressing the psychosocial aspects of breast health, healthcare providers can promote resilience, coping strategies, and quality of life among affected individuals.

Furthermore, promoting breast health fosters a culture of empowerment, advocacy, and inclusivity, recognizing that breast health is a shared responsibility across communities and healthcare systems. Educational initiatives, outreach programs, and policy efforts play vital roles in raising awareness, reducing disparities, and promoting equitable access to breast health services. By prioritizing prevention, early detection, and comprehensive care, stakeholders can work collaboratively to address the multifaceted challenges of breast health and cancer awareness.

CHAPTER THREE

RISK FACTORS FOR BREAST CANCER

Breast cancer is a complex disease influenced by a combination of genetic, environmental, and lifestyle factors. Understanding these risk factors is crucial for early detection, prevention strategies, and personalized healthcare interventions. While some risk factors are beyond individual control, others can be modified through proactive measures, empowering individuals to mitigate their risk and promote breast health.

One of the most well-established risk factors for breast cancer is age. Advancing age is associated with an increased likelihood of developing breast cancer, with the majority of cases diagnosed in women over the age of 50. This highlights the importance of regular screening and vigilance as individuals age, as early detection becomes increasingly critical for favorable outcomes.

Another significant risk factor is genetic predisposition, particularly mutations in the BRCA1 and BRCA2 genes. Inherited mutations in these genes significantly elevate the risk of developing breast and ovarian cancers. Additionally, other genetic variants and family history of breast cancer can also contribute to increased susceptibility. Genetic counseling and testing can help individuals assess their risk and make informed decisions about surveillance and preventive measures.

Hormonal factors play a pivotal role in breast cancer development, with exposure to estrogen and progesterone influencing risk. Early menarche (onset of menstruation), late menopause, and hormone replacement therapy are associated with higher breast cancer risk due to prolonged exposure to estrogen. Similarly, nulliparity (never giving birth) or late age at first childbirth can elevate risk, while breastfeeding has a protective effect by reducing lifetime estrogen exposure.

Furthermore, lifestyle factors such as alcohol consumption, tobacco use, and sedentary behavior can impact breast cancer risk. Excessive alcohol consumption has been linked to increased risk, with even moderate alcohol intake contributing to elevated susceptibility. Conversely, regular physical activity is associated with lower risk, potentially through its effects on hormone metabolism, immune function, and body weight regulation.

Obesity and poor dietary habits are also significant contributors to breast cancer risk. Excess body weight, particularly after menopause, is associated with elevated estrogen levels and chronic inflammation, both of which can promote tumor growth. Consuming a diet rich in fruits, vegetables, whole grains, and lean proteins may help mitigate risk by providing essential nutrients and antioxidants while reducing exposure to potentially carcinogenic substances.

Environmental factors such as exposure to ionizing radiation, certain chemicals, and pollution may also influence breast cancer risk, although their precise impact remains under investigation. Additionally, socioeconomic factors, including access to healthcare, education, and socioeconomic status, can affect breast cancer incidence and outcomes, highlighting the importance of addressing disparities in breast health care.

CHAPTER FOUR

EARLY DETECTION AND SCREENING GUIDELINES

Early detection is a cornerstone of breast cancer management, offering the best chance for successful treatment and improved outcomes. Screening guidelines aim to detect breast cancer in its earliest stages when it is most treatable, often before symptoms manifest. Several screening modalities are available, each with its own benefits and considerations, empowering individuals to make informed decisions about their breast health.

4.1 Mammograms

Mammography is the most widely utilized screening tool for breast cancer and is recommended for women starting at age 40 by many health organizations, including the American Cancer Society and the U.S. Preventive Services Task Force. Mammograms use low-dose X-rays to capture images of breast tissue, allowing radiologists to detect abnormalities such as masses, calcifications, or architectural distortions. While mammography has been instrumental in reducing breast cancer mortality rates, it may have limitations, particularly in women with dense breast tissue, where cancers can be more challenging to detect.

4.2 MRI Screening

Magnetic Resonance Imaging (MRI) is a supplemental screening modality recommended for women at high risk of developing breast cancer, such as those with BRCA1 or BRCA2 mutations or a strong family history of the disease. MRI offers enhanced sensitivity for detecting breast cancer, particularly in dense breast tissue, and can identify lesions that may be missed on mammography. However, MRI screening is more expensive, time-consuming, and may lead to increased rates of false positives, necessitating additional testing and anxiety for patients.

4.3 Breast Self-Exams

Breast self-exams involve individuals examining their breasts regularly to detect any changes or abnormalities. While breast self-exams were previously advocated as a routine screening method, their role in detecting early-stage breast cancer has become more controversial in recent years. Studies have shown that breast self-exams may lead to increased anxiety and unnecessary biopsies without a significant improvement in breast cancer outcomes. However, some organizations still recommend breast self-exams as part of breast health awareness and self-awareness efforts.

4.4 Clinical Breast Exams

Clinical breast exams are physical examinations of the breasts performed by healthcare professionals, typically during routine healthcare visits. These exams complement screening mammograms and can help detect palpable abnormalities or changes in breast tissue. While clinical breast exams may identify concerning findings that warrant further evaluation, they are not as sensitive as imaging modalities like mammography or MRI for detecting early-stage breast cancer.

4.5 Other Screening Methods

In addition to mammography, MRI, breast self-exams, and clinical breast exams, other screening methods are being explored to improve early detection of breast cancer. These include digital breast tomosynthesis (3D mammography), automated whole breast ultrasound, molecular breast imaging, and circulating tumor DNA tests. These emerging technologies hold promise for enhancing breast cancer detection, particularly in women with dense breast tissue or those at high risk of developing the disease.

CHAPTER FIVE

SIGNS AND SYMPTOMS OF BREAST CANCER

Breast cancer is a heterogeneous disease that can manifest in various forms, with symptoms ranging from subtle changes to more noticeable signs. Recognizing these signs and symptoms is essential for early detection, prompt diagnosis, and timely initiation of treatment, all of which are critical factors in improving breast cancer outcomes.

One of the most common signs of breast cancer is the presence of a lump or mass in the breast or underarm area. These lumps may feel firm, irregular in shape, and may or may not be painful. While most breast lumps are benign, any new lump or mass should be evaluated by a healthcare professional to rule out the possibility of cancer. It's important to note that not all breast cancers present as lumps, and other symptoms should also be considered.

Changes in breast size, shape, or contour can also be indicative of breast cancer.

Dimpling, puckering, or indentation of the skin, sometimes resembling the texture of an orange peel, may occur due to underlying tumors pulling on the breast tissue. Additionally, changes in the appearance or texture of the skin, such as redness, scaliness, or thickening, may signal the presence of an underlying malignancy.

Nipple changes are another potential indicator of breast cancer. This can include nipple retraction or inversion, where the nipple, which previously protruded outward, becomes inverted or pulled inward. Discharge from the nipple, particularly if it is bloody, clear, or occurs spontaneously, should also be evaluated by a healthcare provider. Changes in nipple appearance or function may be caused by tumors affecting the underlying breast tissue or ducts.

Breast pain or discomfort is a symptom that can occur in breast cancer, although it is more commonly associated with benign conditions such as fibrocystic changes or hormonal fluctuations. Persistent, unexplained breast pain or discomfort should be evaluated to determine the underlying cause, as it may warrant further investigation.

Swelling, inflammation, or irritation of the breast tissue may occur in some cases of breast cancer, particularly inflammatory breast cancer (IBC). IBC is a rare and aggressive form of breast cancer characterized by rapid onset of symptoms, including redness, warmth, and swelling of the breast. These symptoms can mimic those of an infection, leading to delays in diagnosis and treatment.

Changes in the appearance or texture of the breast skin, such as dimpling, puckering, or thickening, may also indicate the presence of breast cancer. These changes can occur due to the infiltration of cancer cells into the surrounding tissue, disrupting the normal architecture of the breast.

Additionally, unexplained weight loss, fatigue, or persistent cough may be signs of advanced breast cancer that has spread to other parts of the body, such as the lungs or bones. These symptoms may occur as a result of cancer-related metabolic changes, immune system activation, or organ dysfunction.

It's important to emphasize that experiencing one or more of these signs or symptoms does not necessarily mean a person has breast cancer. Many benign conditions can cause similar changes in the breast, and further evaluation by a healthcare professional is needed to determine the underlying cause. However, any persistent or concerning symptoms should prompt prompt medical attention and evaluation to ensure timely diagnosis and appropriate management.

Recognizing the signs and symptoms of breast cancer is crucial for early detection and timely intervention. By being aware of changes in breast appearance, texture, or function, individuals can take proactive steps to seek medical evaluation and pursue appropriate screening and diagnostic tests. Through increased awareness, education, and advocacy, efforts can be made to improve breast cancer outcomes and reduce the burden of this disease on individuals and communities worldwide.

CHAPTER SIX

DIAGNOSIS AND STAGING

Diagnosing breast cancer involves a comprehensive evaluation of clinical findings, imaging studies, and tissue analysis to confirm the presence of cancerous cells and determine the extent of disease spread. This process is essential for guiding treatment decisions and developing personalized care plans tailored to individual patient needs.

6.1 Biopsy Procedures

Biopsy procedures are the gold standard for diagnosing breast cancer, allowing healthcare providers to obtain tissue samples for laboratory analysis. There are several types of biopsy procedures, including:

Core Needle Biopsy: In this minimally invasive procedure, a hollow needle is used to extract small tissue samples from the suspicious area in the breast. Core needle biopsies are typically performed under local anesthesia and may be guided by imaging techniques such as mammography, ultrasound, or MRI.

Fine Needle Aspiration (FNA): FNA involves using a thin needle to withdraw fluid or tissue from a breast lump or lymph node. This technique is often used to evaluate cysts or to sample suspicious areas identified on imaging studies.

Surgical Biopsy: In cases where core needle biopsy or FNA is inconclusive or not feasible, a surgical biopsy may be performed. This involves removing a larger tissue sample through a surgical incision under general anesthesia. Surgical biopsies may be excisional (removing the entire tumor) or incisional (removing a portion of the tumor for analysis).

After obtaining tissue samples, pathologists analyze the specimens under a microscope to determine whether cancerous cells are present, and if so, to characterize the type, grade, and other molecular features of the tumor. This information is essential for determining the appropriate treatment approach and predicting prognosis.

6.2 Imaging Tests

Imaging tests are essential for assessing the extent of disease and identifying potential sites of cancer spread. Several imaging modalities may be used in the diagnosis and staging of breast cancer, including:

Mammography: Mammography is a standard imaging test used for breast cancer screening and diagnosis. It involves taking X-ray images of the breast tissue to detect abnormalities such as masses, calcifications, or architectural distortions. Mammography is particularly useful for identifying early-stage breast cancer before it becomes symptomatic.

Ultrasound: Breast ultrasound uses sound waves to produce images of the breast tissue. It is often used as a supplemental imaging tool to evaluate suspicious areas identified on mammography or to distinguish between solid and cystic lesions. Ultrasound is helpful for guiding biopsy procedures and assessing lymph node involvement.

Magnetic Resonance Imaging (MRI): Breast MRI is a highly sensitive imaging modality that uses magnetic fields and radio waves to create detailed images of the breast tissue. It is particularly useful for evaluating the extent of disease in the breast, detecting multifocal or multicentric tumors, and assessing tumor response to neoadjuvant therapy.

6.3 Staging of Breast Cancer

Once breast cancer is diagnosed, healthcare providers use a staging system to determine the extent of disease spread and guide treatment decisions. The most commonly used staging system for breast cancer is the TNM system, which classifies tumors based on the size of the primary tumor (T), the involvement of nearby lymph nodes (N), and the presence of distant metastases (M).

Staging helps healthcare providers categorize breast cancer into different stages (0 through IV) based on tumor size, lymph node involvement, and distant metastases. This information helps predict prognosis and guides treatment decisions, with earlier-stage cancers generally associated with better outcomes.

CHAPTER SEVEN

TREATMENT OPTIONS

Treatment options for various medical conditions have evolved significantly over the years, offering patients a range of interventions tailored to their specific needs. Among these options, surgery, radiation therapy, chemotherapy, hormonal therapy, and targeted therapy stand as prominent pillars in the fight against numerous ailments, including cancer. Each modality presents distinct mechanisms and benefits, contributing to the comprehensive approach in managing diseases.

7.1 Surgery

Surgery remains a cornerstone in the treatment of many conditions, particularly cancer. It involves the physical removal of tumors or diseased tissue from the body. Surgeons employ various techniques, including traditional open surgery, minimally invasive procedures like laparoscopy, and robotic-assisted surgeries for enhanced precision. The primary goal of surgery is to excise localized tumors, prevent their spread, and alleviate symptoms. Despite its invasiveness, surgery offers the potential for a cure, especially when tumors are detected early and confined to a specific area.

7.2 Radiation Therapy

Radiation therapy utilizes high-energy radiation to target and destroy cancer cells. It can be delivered externally (external beam radiation) or internally (brachytherapy), depending on the tumor's location and type. By damaging the DNA within cancer cells, radiation therapy impedes their ability to multiply and grow. This treatment is often used in conjunction with surgery or chemotherapy to shrink tumors before surgical removal or to eradicate remaining cancer cells post-surgery. Radiation therapy is also effective in palliating symptoms, such as pain or obstruction, improving patients' quality of life.

7.3 Chemotherapy

Chemotherapy involves the use of powerful drugs to kill rapidly dividing cells, including cancer cells. These drugs can be administered orally, intravenously, or via injection, allowing for systemic distribution throughout the body. Chemotherapy is particularly beneficial in treating cancers that have spread extensively or those that are inherently sensitive to certain drugs. While chemotherapy can cause side effects due to its impact on healthy cells, such as hair loss and nausea, advances in drug development have led to the emergence of more targeted and tolerable regimens.

7.4 Hormonal Therapy

Hormonal therapy, also known as endocrine therapy, is employed in the management of hormone-sensitive cancers, such as breast and prostate cancer. It works by blocking or inhibiting the body's production of certain hormones or by interfering with hormone receptors on cancer cells. By depriving tumors of the hormones they need to grow, hormonal therapy can slow cancer progression and alleviate symptoms. This treatment is often well-tolerated with fewer side effects compared to chemotherapy, making it a favorable option for certain patients.

7.5 Targeted Therapy

Targeted therapy involves the use of drugs or other substances to specifically target cancer cells while minimizing damage to healthy tissue. Unlike chemotherapy, which affects all rapidly dividing cells, targeted therapy exploits unique molecular characteristics or pathways present in cancer cells. By honing in on these specific targets, targeted therapy can disrupt cancer cell growth and survival more selectively. This approach has led to significant advancements in precision medicine, allowing for tailored treatment strategies based on individual tumor profiles and genetic mutations.

CHAPTER EIGHT

SURVIVORSHIP AND SUPPORTIVE CARE

Survivorship and supportive care play crucial roles in the comprehensive management of individuals affected by breast cancer, ensuring that patients receive holistic support throughout their journey from diagnosis to long-term recovery. As advancements in breast cancer treatment have improved survival rates, there is an increasing focus on addressing the physical, emotional, and psychosocial needs of breast cancer survivors and their caregivers.

Survivorship encompasses the period following cancer treatment, which may last for many years or even a lifetime. During this phase, survivors often face various challenges related to physical health, emotional well-being, social relationships, and practical concerns such as employment and financial stability. Supportive care aims to address these challenges through a multidisciplinary approach that addresses the diverse needs of survivors and promotes their overall well-being.

Physical Health:

Cancer survivors may experience long-term or late effects of treatment, such as fatigue, pain, neuropathy, lymphedema, and cognitive changes. Survivorship care includes regular monitoring for these potential side effects and providing interventions to manage symptoms and improve quality of life. Rehabilitation services, physical therapy, and integrative therapies such as yoga and acupuncture may also be beneficial in addressing physical issues.

Emotional Well-being:

The emotional impact of cancer diagnosis and treatment can be profound, leading to feelings of anxiety, depression, fear of recurrence, and post-traumatic stress. Survivorship programs offer counseling, support groups, and psychiatric services to help survivors cope with these emotional challenges. Psychosocial support aims to improve resilience, promote self-care strategies, and enhance coping skills to navigate the emotional ups and downs of survivorship.

Social Support:

Maintaining social connections and support networks is essential for cancer survivors as they transition back to their daily lives. Supportive care programs facilitate peer support groups, educational workshops, and community resources to foster social connections and reduce feelings of isolation. Addressing issues related to family dynamics, communication, and caregiver support is also integral to the overall well-being of survivors and their loved ones.

Practical Concerns:

Cancer survivors may encounter practical challenges related to employment, insurance, finances, and access to healthcare services. Survivorship programs offer resources and guidance to address these practical concerns, including assistance with navigating insurance coverage, accessing financial support programs, and transitioning back to work or school after treatment.

CHAPTER NINE

LIFESTYLE FACTORS FOR BREAST HEALTH

Maintaining breast health is crucial for preventing breast cancer and promoting overall well-being. Lifestyle factors, including diet and nutrition, exercise and physical activity, as well as smoking and alcohol consumption, play significant roles in breast health. Adopting healthy habits in these areas can reduce the risk of developing breast cancer and contribute to better breast health outcomes.

9.1 Diet and Nutrition

A balanced diet rich in fruits, vegetables, whole grains, lean proteins, and healthy fats can support breast health by providing essential nutrients and antioxidants. Research suggests that certain dietary factors may influence breast cancer risk. For instance, consuming a diet high in fruits and vegetables, particularly cruciferous vegetables like broccoli and kale, may help reduce the risk of breast cancer due to their anti-inflammatory and antioxidant properties. Additionally, incorporating omega-3 fatty acids from sources such as fatty fish, flaxseeds, and walnuts may have protective effects against breast cancer development. Conversely, a diet high in processed foods, sugary beverages, and saturated fats may increase the risk of breast cancer and other chronic diseases. Limiting intake of red and processed meats, sugary snacks, and refined carbohydrates can contribute to overall breast health.

9.2 Exercise and Physical Activity

Regular exercise and physical activity are associated with numerous health benefits, including reduced risk of breast cancer and improved breast health. Engaging in moderate-intensity aerobic activities such as brisk walking, jogging, cycling, or swimming for at least 150 minutes per week can help maintain a healthy weight and lower estrogen levels, which may decrease the risk of hormone receptor-positive breast cancer. Strength training exercises that target the chest, back, and arm muscles can also help improve breast health by supporting overall muscle tone and posture.

Additionally, regular physical activity has been shown to reduce inflammation, enhance immune function, and improve mood and sleep quality, all of which contribute to better breast health outcomes.

9.3 Smoking and Alcohol Consumption

Smoking and excessive alcohol consumption are established risk factors for various cancers, including breast cancer. Tobacco smoke contains carcinogens that can damage DNA and increase the risk of cancer development, including breast cancer. Therefore, quitting smoking or avoiding exposure to secondhand smoke is essential for maintaining breast health and reducing cancer risk. Similarly, alcohol consumption, particularly heavy drinking, is associated with an increased risk of breast cancer. Alcohol can raise estrogen levels in the body, which may promote the growth of hormone receptor-positive breast cancer cells. Limiting alcohol intake to no more than one drink per day for women and avoiding binge drinking can help lower breast cancer risk and promote overall health.

CHAPTER TEN

GENETIC FACTORS AND FAMILY HISTORY

Genetic factors and family history play significant roles in determining an individual's risk of developing various health conditions, including breast cancer. Understanding one's genetic predisposition and family history of breast cancer is essential for early detection, prevention, and personalized risk management strategies.

Genetic Factors:

Certain genetic mutations can increase the risk of breast cancer. The most well-known genes associated with hereditary breast cancer are BRCA1 and BRCA2. Mutations in these genes significantly elevate the lifetime risk of developing breast and ovarian cancers, as well as other cancers such as prostate and pancreatic cancer. Other less common genetic mutations, such as TP53 (associated with Li-Fraumeni syndrome), PTEN (associated with Cowden syndrome), and PALB2, also contribute to an increased risk of breast cancer. Genetic testing can identify these mutations and provide valuable information about an individual's cancer risk. For individuals with known genetic mutations, proactive measures such as increased surveillance, risk-reducing surgeries, and chemoprevention strategies may be recommended to mitigate the risk of developing breast cancer.

Family History:

A family history of breast cancer can also influence an individual's risk of developing the disease. Having a first-degree relative (parent, sibling, or child) with breast cancer doubles the risk of developing breast cancer compared to individuals without a family history. Additionally, having multiple relatives affected by breast cancer, particularly at a young age, or a family history of ovarian cancer, may further elevate the risk. It's important to note that while genetic factors contribute to a small percentage of breast cancer cases, the majority of cases occur sporadically and are not directly attributable to inherited genetic mutations. Nevertheless, individuals with a strong family history of breast cancer may benefit from genetic counseling and testing to assess their risk and develop personalized risk management plans.

Early detection and risk reduction strategies are critical for individuals with genetic predispositions or family histories of breast cancer. Screening guidelines may be tailored based on individual risk factors, including earlier initiation of mammography and consideration of additional screening modalities such as breast MRI. Risk-reducing strategies may include lifestyle modifications, chemoprevention with medications such as tamoxifen or aromatase inhibitors, and risk-reducing surgeries such as prophylactic mastectomy or oophorectomy for individuals with high-risk genetic mutations.

CHAPTER ELEVEN

EMOTIONAL AND PSYCHOLOGICAL IMPACT OF BREAST CANCER

The emotional and psychological impact of breast cancer can be profound and far-reaching, affecting individuals diagnosed with the disease, as well as their loved ones and caregivers. Coping with a breast cancer diagnosis involves navigating a wide range of emotions, including fear, anxiety, sadness, anger, and uncertainty. Understanding and addressing these emotional challenges are essential components of comprehensive cancer care, as they can significantly impact a patient's quality of life and overall well-being.

Diagnosis and Treatment Shock:

Receiving a breast cancer diagnosis can be overwhelming and shocking, often leading to a whirlwind of emotions for patients and their families. The news of a cancer diagnosis may evoke feelings of disbelief, fear of the unknown, and a sense of vulnerability. Coping with the physical and emotional demands of treatment, such as surgery, chemotherapy, radiation therapy, and hormonal therapy, further adds to the emotional burden. Patients may experience distressing symptoms, such as pain, fatigue, hair loss, and changes in body image, which can exacerbate feelings of distress and anxiety.

Fear of Recurrence:

Even after completing treatment and achieving remission, many breast cancer survivors grapple with the persistent fear of cancer recurrence. The uncertainty about the future and the possibility of cancer returning can lead to heightened anxiety, hypervigilance, and intrusive thoughts. Coping with the fear of recurrence requires ongoing support, coping strategies, and a sense of empowerment to navigate life after cancer with resilience and optimism.

Body Image and Self-Esteem:

Breast cancer and its treatment can profoundly impact a woman's body image and sense of femininity. Surgical procedures such as mastectomy, lumpectomy, and reconstruction may alter the appearance of the breasts, leading to feelings of disfigurement, loss of identity, and diminished self-esteem. Coping with changes in physical appearance and reclaiming a positive body image often require emotional support, counseling, and self-care practices to foster acceptance, self-love, and empowerment.

Relationships and Social Support:

Breast cancer can strain relationships with partners, family members, and friends, as patients and caregivers navigate the challenges of diagnosis, treatment, and recovery. Communication breakdowns, role changes, and caregiving responsibilities may create tension and conflict within relationships. However, strong social support networks, open communication, and empathy can foster resilience, strengthen relationships, and provide emotional sustenance during difficult times.

Psychosocial Support and Coping Strategies:

Addressing the emotional and psychological impact of breast cancer requires a multidisciplinary approach that integrates psychosocial support services, counseling, and coping strategies. Support groups, individual counseling, mindfulness-based therapies, art therapy, and relaxation techniques can help patients cope with stress, manage emotional distress, and cultivate resilience. Encouraging self-care practices, engaging in meaningful activities, and fostering a sense of purpose and hope are essential components of psychosocial support for breast cancer patients and survivors.

CHAPTER TWELVE

CLINICAL TRIALS AND EMERGING RESEARCH

Clinical trials and emerging research play pivotal roles in advancing our understanding of breast cancer, improving treatment outcomes, and ultimately finding a cure for the disease. These studies contribute to the development of new therapies, diagnostic tools, and prevention strategies, offering hope for better outcomes and quality of life for breast cancer patients and survivors.

Drug Development and Treatment Innovation:

Clinical trials are instrumental in evaluating the safety and efficacy of novel drugs and treatment modalities for breast cancer. These studies assess new targeted therapies, immunotherapies, and combination treatments designed to inhibit cancer growth, improve survival rates, and minimize side effects. By participating in clinical trials, patients have access to cutting-edge treatments that may not be available through standard care, potentially offering them better outcomes and quality of life. Recent advancements in precision medicine have led to the development of targeted therapies that exploit specific molecular pathways and genetic mutations driving breast cancer, such as HER2-targeted therapies and PARP inhibitors.

Personalized Medicine and Biomarker Discovery:

Emerging research in genomics, proteomics, and molecular profiling is revolutionizing the field of breast cancer treatment by enabling personalized medicine approaches. By analyzing the genetic and molecular characteristics of individual tumors, researchers can identify biomarkers that predict treatment response, disease progression, and prognosis. Biomarker-driven clinical trials aim to match patients with targeted therapies based on their tumor's unique molecular profile, maximizing treatment efficacy and minimizing unnecessary toxicity. Examples of biomarkers used in breast cancer research include hormone receptors (estrogen receptor, progesterone receptor), HER2 status, and genetic mutations (BRCA1, BRCA2).

Immunotherapy and Immunogenomics:

Immunotherapy has emerged as a promising treatment modality for breast cancer, harnessing the body's immune system to recognize and destroy cancer cells. Clinical trials are investigating immune checkpoint inhibitors, chimeric antigen receptor (CAR) T-cell therapy, cancer vaccines, and adoptive cell therapy in various breast cancer subtypes. Additionally, research in immunogenomics aims to elucidate the complex interplay between the tumor microenvironment, immune response, and tumor progression, offering insights into novel therapeutic targets and combination strategies to enhance immunotherapy efficacy.

Prevention and Early Detection:

Clinical trials are exploring innovative approaches to breast cancer prevention and early detection, including chemoprevention agents, lifestyle interventions, and novel imaging technologies. These studies aim to identify high-risk individuals, reduce the incidence of breast cancer, and improve screening methods for early disease detection. Research in breast cancer risk assessment models, genetic testing, and breast density evaluation is enhancing our ability to identify individuals at increased risk and tailor preventive strategies accordingly.

CHAPTER THIRTEEN

ADVOCACY AND AWARENESS EFFORTS

Advocacy and awareness efforts are essential components of the global fight against breast cancer, empowering individuals, communities, and policymakers to take action, promote early detection, and support those affected by the disease. Through education, advocacy campaigns, fundraising initiatives, and policy advocacy, advocates strive to raise awareness about breast cancer risk factors, screening guidelines, treatment options, and survivorship issues, ultimately improving outcomes and reducing the burden of breast cancer worldwide.

Education and Outreach:

Advocacy organizations and healthcare institutions play a crucial role in educating the public about breast cancer prevention, early detection, and treatment. Through community outreach programs, workshops, educational materials, and online resources, advocates disseminate evidence-based information about breast health, risk factors, and screening guidelines. By empowering individuals with knowledge and awareness, advocacy efforts aim to promote proactive health behaviors, encourage regular breast self-exams and clinical breast exams, and increase participation in mammography screening programs.

Empowerment and Support:

Breast cancer advocacy is grounded in the principles of empowerment, support, and solidarity for individuals affected by the disease. Advocacy organizations provide a wide range of support services, including peer support groups, counseling, financial assistance, and access to resources for patients, survivors, and caregivers. By fostering a sense of community, advocacy efforts empower individuals to navigate the challenges of diagnosis, treatment, and survivorship with resilience, hope, and dignity.

Policy Advocacy and Research Funding:

Advocates work tirelessly to influence public policy, secure funding for breast cancer research, and advocate for legislative measures that promote access to quality healthcare, cancer screenings, and treatment services. Through grassroots advocacy campaigns, lobbying efforts, and collaboration with policymakers, advocates advocate for increased funding for breast cancer research, improved insurance coverage for screening and treatment, and policies that prioritize patient-centered care, survivorship support, and equitable access to healthcare services.

Cultural Competence and Health Equity:

Breast cancer advocacy efforts recognize the importance of cultural competence and health equity in addressing disparities in breast cancer outcomes among diverse populations. Advocates work to raise awareness about the unique challenges faced by underserved communities, including racial and ethnic minorities, low-income individuals, LGBTQ+ individuals, and rural populations. By promoting culturally sensitive outreach, language-accessible resources, and targeted interventions, advocates strive to eliminate barriers to breast cancer screening, diagnosis, and treatment and improve health outcomes for all.

Global Collaboration and Impact:

Breast cancer advocacy is a global movement that transcends borders, uniting individuals, organizations, and governments in the shared mission of ending breast cancer. International partnerships, collaborative research efforts, and advocacy networks facilitate the exchange of knowledge, resources, and best practices to address the global burden of breast cancer and improve access to quality care and treatment services in low-resource settings.

CHAPTER FOURTEEN

RESOURCES FOR PATIENTS AND CAREGIVERS

Navigating a breast cancer diagnosis can be overwhelming for patients and their caregivers, but numerous resources are available to provide support, information, and assistance throughout the journey. From support organizations and online communities to financial assistance programs, these resources offer valuable support and guidance to individuals affected by breast cancer.

14.1 Support Organizations

Support organizations play a crucial role in providing emotional support, practical assistance, and educational resources to breast cancer patients and their families. These organizations offer a wide range of services, including peer support groups, counseling services, helplines, and educational workshops. Organizations such as the American Cancer Society, Susan G. Komen for the Cure, Breast Cancer Network of Strength, and Living Beyond Breast

Cancer provide comprehensive support services tailored to the needs of breast cancer patients and survivors. These organizations also advocate for policies that prioritize breast cancer research, access to quality care, and patient-centered support services.

14.2 Online Communities

Online communities and forums provide a platform for breast cancer patients and caregivers to connect, share experiences, and seek advice from others who have been through similar challenges. Websites such as Breastcancer.org, Inspire, and MyBCTeam offer virtual support networks where individuals can join discussion groups, ask questions, and access educational resources. Online communities provide a sense of belonging, validation, and empowerment for individuals facing a breast cancer diagnosis, allowing them to find camaraderie and support from the comfort of their own homes.

14.3 Financial Assistance Programs

Financial concerns can add additional stress to the already challenging experience of dealing with breast cancer. Fortunately, there are numerous financial assistance programs available to help alleviate the financial burden associated with medical expenses, treatment costs, and other related expenses. Organizations such as the Patient Advocate Foundation, CancerCare, and the Pink Fund offer financial assistance programs that provide grants, co-payment assistance, transportation assistance, and help with other practical needs. These programs aim to ensure that patients have access to the care and support they need without facing undue financial hardship.

CHAPTER FIFTEEN

INTEGRATIVE MEDICINE AND COMPLEMENTARY THERAPIES

Integrative medicine and complementary therapies have gained recognition as valuable adjuncts to conventional cancer treatment, including breast cancer care. These approaches focus on addressing the physical, emotional, and spiritual aspects of healing, enhancing quality of life, and promoting overall well-being for breast cancer patients. By integrating evidence-based complementary therapies with standard medical care, patients can experience a more comprehensive and holistic approach to managing the challenges of cancer diagnosis, treatment, and survivorship.

Mind-Body Practices:

Mind-body practices such as meditation, mindfulness, yoga, and tai chi offer profound benefits for breast cancer patients by promoting relaxation, stress reduction, and emotional resilience. These practices help patients cope with the psychological and emotional distress associated with cancer diagnosis and treatment, reducing anxiety, depression, and fatigue. Mindfulness-based stress reduction (MBSR) programs, in particular, have been shown to improve mood, decrease pain, and enhance quality of life for breast cancer patients undergoing treatment.

Acupuncture and Traditional Chinese Medicine:

Acupuncture, an ancient practice rooted in Traditional Chinese Medicine (TCM), involves the insertion of thin needles into specific points on the body to stimulate healing and restore balance. For breast cancer patients, acupuncture can help alleviate treatment-related symptoms such as nausea, pain, hot flashes, neuropathy, and fatigue. Additionally, TCM modalities such as herbal medicine, moxibustion, and dietary therapy may complement conventional treatment approaches and support overall health and well-being.

Nutritional Therapy:

Nutritional therapy plays a vital role in supporting breast cancer patients' overall health and optimizing treatment outcomes.

A well-balanced diet rich in fruits, vegetables, whole grains, lean proteins, and healthy fats can help bolster the immune system, reduce inflammation, and promote healing. Integrative nutrition counseling and dietary supplements may also be beneficial in addressing specific nutritional needs, managing treatment side effects, and supporting overall wellness during and after breast cancer treatment.

Physical Therapy and Exercise:

Physical therapy and exercise programs tailored to the unique needs of breast cancer patients can help improve physical function, alleviate treatment-related side effects, and enhance quality of life. Exercise has been shown to reduce fatigue, improve strength and mobility, boost mood, and lower the risk of cancer recurrence. Integrative physical therapy approaches, such as lymphedema management, scar tissue mobilization, and gentle stretching exercises, can help patients regain function and vitality after surgery or radiation therapy.

Psychosocial Support and Counseling:

Psychosocial support and counseling services are integral components of integrative cancer care, providing emotional support, coping strategies, and therapeutic interventions to address the psychological and emotional challenges of breast cancer. Individual counseling, support groups, art therapy, and expressive arts modalities can help patients process their feelings, cope with stress, and find meaning and purpose in their cancer journey.

CHAPTER SIXTEEN

FERTILITY PRESERVATION AND BREAST CANCER

For many women diagnosed with breast cancer, concerns about fertility preservation are paramount. Breast cancer treatments such as chemotherapy, radiation therapy, and hormonal therapy can potentially impact fertility, leading to temporary or permanent infertility. However, advancements in fertility preservation techniques offer hope for women seeking to preserve their fertility before undergoing breast cancer treatment.

Fertility Preservation Options:

There are several fertility preservation options available to women diagnosed with breast cancer. One common method is cryopreservation of embryos, where eggs are retrieved from the ovaries, fertilized with sperm in a laboratory, and then frozen for later use. Another option is oocyte cryopreservation, where eggs are retrieved and frozen without fertilization. Additionally, ovarian tissue cryopreservation involves removing and freezing ovarian tissue, which can later be transplanted back into the woman's body to restore ovarian function. These fertility preservation techniques allow women to retain the option of having biological children in the future after completing breast cancer treatment.

Timing of Fertility Preservation:

The timing of fertility preservation is crucial for women diagnosed with breast cancer, as treatment may need to be initiated promptly to prevent disease progression. Ideally, discussions about fertility preservation should occur as soon as possible after diagnosis to allow for timely decision-making and initiation of fertility preservation procedures before starting cancer treatment. However, in some cases, fertility preservation may need to be delayed due to the urgency of starting cancer treatment or concerns about treatment delays impacting prognosis.

Multidisciplinary Collaboration:

Multidisciplinary collaboration between oncologists, fertility specialists, and reproductive endocrinologists is essential in providing comprehensive care for women with breast cancer who are considering fertility preservation. Oncologists can provide information about the potential impact of cancer treatment on fertility and help weigh the risks and benefits of delaying treatment for fertility preservation. Fertility specialists can discuss available fertility preservation options, assess ovarian reserve, and facilitate fertility preservation procedures. Collaboration between these healthcare providers ensures that women receive individualized care that addresses both their oncological and reproductive needs.

Supportive Care and Counseling:

Supportive care and counseling play integral roles in helping women navigate the complex emotional and practical considerations associated with fertility preservation and breast cancer treatment. Fertility preservation decisions can be emotionally challenging, and women may benefit from counseling to explore their feelings, concerns, and priorities regarding fertility and family-building options. Additionally, support groups and peer counseling can provide women with opportunities to connect with others who have faced similar challenges and share experiences and coping strategies.

CHAPTER SEVENTEEN

BREAST RECONSTRUCTION OPTIONS

Breast reconstruction is an important aspect of breast cancer treatment for many women who undergo mastectomy or lumpectomy. Reconstruction can help restore a sense of wholeness, body image, and self-confidence following breast cancer surgery. There are several options available for breast reconstruction, each with its own advantages, considerations, and potential outcomes.

Implant-Based Reconstruction:

Implant-based reconstruction involves the use of saline or silicone implants to recreate the shape and volume of the breast. This approach may be performed either immediately following mastectomy (immediate reconstruction) or as a separate procedure after mastectomy and completion of cancer treatment (delayed reconstruction). Implant-based reconstruction offers a relatively straightforward surgical procedure, shorter recovery time, and minimal scarring compared to autologous tissue reconstruction. However, it may require additional surgeries for implant adjustments, replacements, or revisions over time, and there is a risk of complications such as capsular contracture or implant rupture.

Autologous Tissue Reconstruction:

Autologous tissue reconstruction, also known as flap reconstruction, involves using the patient's own tissue from another part of the body to create a new breast mound. Common donor sites for autologous tissue include the abdomen (TRAM flap or DIEP flap), back (latissimus dorsi flap), or buttocks (gluteal flap). Flap reconstruction offers a more natural look and feel compared to implants, as the reconstructed breast tissue is made from the patient's own body. However, flap reconstruction is a more complex surgical procedure with longer recovery time, and it may result in additional scars and donor site morbidity. It also requires sufficient donor tissue and may not be suitable for all patients.

Combination Approaches:

Some women may benefit from a combination of implant-based reconstruction and autologous tissue reconstruction, known as hybrid or staged reconstruction. This approach allows for the advantages of both techniques, such as the initial placement of tissue expanders or implants followed by later conversion to autologous tissue reconstruction for improved aesthetics and long-term outcomes.

CHAPTER EIGHTEEN

SUPPORT GROUPS AND PEER NETWORKS

Support groups and peer networks play invaluable roles in providing emotional support, information, and camaraderie for individuals affected by breast cancer. These groups offer safe spaces where patients, survivors, and caregivers can share their experiences, fears, and triumphs with others who understand their journey firsthand.

Participating in support groups allows individuals to connect with others facing similar challenges, providing a sense of belonging and validation. Through shared stories and shared experiences, participants can gain insights, coping strategies, and practical advice for navigating the physical, emotional, and practical aspects of breast cancer diagnosis, treatment, and survivorship.

Support groups offer emotional support, encouragement, and empathy during difficult times, helping individuals feel less isolated and alone in their struggles. Peer networks also provide opportunities for personal growth, empowerment, and advocacy, as participants become advocates for themselves and others affected by breast cancer.

Support groups and peer networks foster a sense of community, resilience, and hope for individuals affected by breast cancer, empowering them to face their challenges with courage, strength, and dignity.

CHAPTER NINETEEN

SURVIVOR STORIES AND INSPIRATIONAL NARRATIVES

Survivor stories and inspirational narratives play powerful roles in providing hope, encouragement, and validation for individuals affected by breast cancer. These stories, shared by survivors, caregivers, and advocates, offer insights into the lived experiences of those who have faced and overcome the challenges of breast cancer diagnosis, treatment, and survivorship.

Survivor stories highlight the resilience, courage, and strength of individuals who have navigated the uncertainties and fears of a breast cancer diagnosis. By sharing their personal journeys, survivors offer hope and inspiration to others facing similar challenges, demonstrating that it is possible to overcome adversity and emerge stronger on the other side.

Inspirational narratives provide comfort and reassurance to individuals grappling with the physical and emotional toll of breast cancer. These stories celebrate the triumphs, milestones, and victories achieved by survivors, reminding others that they are not alone in their struggles and that there is light at the end of the tunnel.

Survivor stories also serve as powerful advocacy tools, raising awareness about breast cancer, promoting early detection, and destigmatizing conversations about the disease. By sharing their stories publicly, survivors help educate others about the importance of self-exams, mammograms, and proactive health behaviors, empowering individuals to take charge of their breast health and seek timely medical care.

Moreover, survivor stories foster a sense of community and solidarity among individuals affected by breast cancer, creating connections and bonds that transcend geographic boundaries and cultural differences. Through shared narratives, survivors find validation, support, and understanding from others who have walked similar paths, fostering a sense of belonging and camaraderie.

CHAPTER TWENTY

CONCLUSION: EMPOWERING BREAST HEALTH

Empowering breast health is a fundamental aspect of comprehensive healthcare, encompassing education, awareness, advocacy, and support initiatives aimed at promoting breast cancer prevention, early detection, and survivorship. By prioritizing breast health at individual, community, and societal levels, we can empower individuals to take proactive steps towards maintaining their breast health and reducing their risk of breast cancer.

Education is key to empowering individuals with the knowledge and tools they need to make informed decisions about their breast health. Providing accurate information about breast cancer risk factors, screening guidelines, and self-examination techniques equips individuals with the awareness and confidence to prioritize their breast health. Educational campaigns, workshops, and outreach programs play vital roles in disseminating this information and raising awareness about the importance of regular breast health screenings and early detection.

Promoting access to breast health services is essential for empowering individuals to take charge of their breast health. This includes ensuring equitable access to mammography screening, clinical breast exams, genetic testing, and other preventive services for all individuals, regardless of socioeconomic status, race, ethnicity, or geographic location. By addressing barriers to care and promoting health equity, we can empower marginalized and underserved communities to prioritize their breast health and seek timely medical intervention when needed.

Advocacy efforts are crucial in driving policy changes and systemic reforms that support breast health empowerment. This includes advocating for legislation that improves access to breast health services, increases funding for breast cancer research, and supports initiatives to reduce environmental risk factors linked to breast cancer development. By amplifying the voices of breast cancer survivors, caregivers, and advocates, we can advocate for policies that prioritize breast health and improve outcomes for individuals affected by breast cancer.

Support services and resources are vital for empowering individuals affected by breast cancer to navigate their journey with dignity, resilience, and hope. This includes providing emotional support, counseling, peer mentoring, and practical assistance to individuals undergoing treatment, as well as survivorship programs and resources for long-term survivors. By fostering a supportive and inclusive community, we can empower individuals to overcome the physical, emotional, and psychological challenges of breast cancer and thrive beyond their diagnosis.

In conclusion, empowering breast health requires a collaborative and multifaceted approach that involves education, advocacy, and support initiatives at individual, community, and societal levels. By prioritizing breast health awareness, promoting access to care, advocating for policy changes, and providing comprehensive support services, we can empower individuals to take control of their breast health and reduce their risk of breast cancer. Together, we can work towards a future where every individual has the knowledge, resources, and support they need to achieve optimal breast health and well-being.

www.ingramcontent.com/pod-product-compliance
Lightning Source LLC
Chambersburg PA
CBHW051650250726

48653CB00007B/2582